AF382202

ESSENTIAL OILS

Reap the benefits of natural remedies

Written by Dominique van der Kaa
Translated by Emma Hanna

Health and Wellbeing 50MINUTES.com

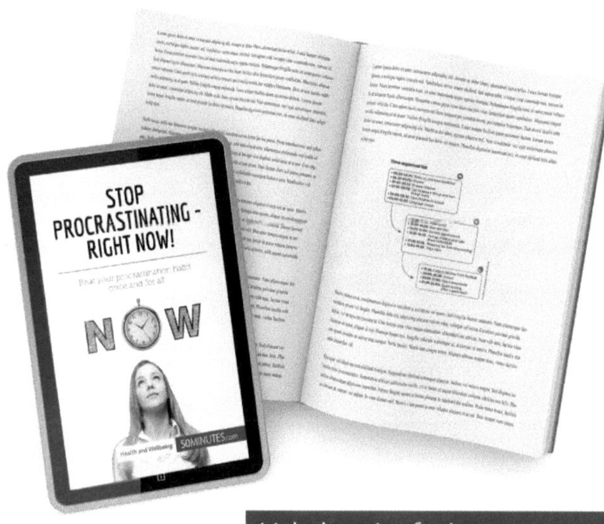

50MINUTES.com

HEALTH AND WELLBEING
WITHOUT THE HEADACHE

STOP PROCRASTINATING - RIGHT NOW!

NOW

Health and Wellbeing
50MINUTES.com

Make learning fun!

Learn to love yourself

Dealing with bullying at school

Your guide to making friends

www.50minutes.com

ESSENTIAL OILS

UNLOCK THEIR NATURAL BENEFITS

- **Problem:** essential oils have a wide variety of properties. Some of them have antiseptic or antimicrobial properties, while others can purify the air or repel insects. They have been used in aromatherapy for millennia and are a natural complement to any kind of therapeutic medicine. They can also be used to give household cleaning products a natural fragrance. Knowing all this, how can we use them effectively?
- **Aim:** to learn about essential oils and how they can be used in aromatherapy and in everyday life to create a cleaner, healthier home environment.
- **FAQs:**
  - How should essential oils be stored?
  - What is the difference between essential oils and vegetable oils?
  - Can essential oils cause allergic reactions?
  - Which essential oil should I buy first?

- How should I react to an accident?
- Where can I buy essential oils?

Essential oils are naturally occurring plant aromas. Since time immemorial, humans have extracted these aromatic active agents to create essential oils and use them to clean or purify our homes. But what are they, how can they be extracted, what can they be used for and what problems or ailments can they alleviate?

In just 50 minutes, you will enter the world of essential oils and discover their various uses, including easing a variety of ailments, clearing your skin, improving your wellbeing and cleaning your house. You will learn about them and the ways you can use them safely at home to create a healthier environment and feel good in your skin.

WARNING

Although self-medication is not recommended and it is important to go through a qualified aromatherapy doctor to obtain your essential oils (especially those designed for oral consumption, given that they are hyperactive and toxic), it is possible to use them yourself as long as you follow a few cautionary guidelines.

- Essential oils should not be used as a substitute for medical treatment and a balanced diet.
- Certain essential oils can cause skin irritation. With a few exceptions, you should never apply pure oils to your skin directly.
- Always wash your hands after use.
- Avoid any contact with your eyes; do not apply essential oils to the ear canal or genital areas.
- Essential oils are insoluble. This means you should never attempt to dilute them in water, as this risks irritating the area around your mouth and preventing you from ingesting enough of them to be beneficial. Similarly, essential oils should never be added to bathwater directly, but should be dissolved

in a hydro-dispersant base such as a neutral shower gel or vegetable oil.

- Never allow children under seven to ingest essential oils orally and always keep them out of the reach of children.
- Always adhere to the dosage, means of consumption and treatment period recommended by your aromatherapist.
- Always use essential oils for a short period of time (three weeks maximum) and leave a week between treatments if necessary.
- Avoid exposure to direct sunlight after applying photosensitive essential oils (generally those extracted from citrus plants).
- Essential oil aerosol sprays should never be used in the presence of children under 30 months; wait 30 minutes before bringing them back into the room where the spray was used. The same rule applies for pregnant women and individuals with asthma or perfume allergies. The room will be mostly aerated once the particles disperse.
- Do not use essential oil diffusers while sleeping, as this risks over-saturating the air and irritating your mucous membranes.
- Avoid using old essential oils (check the expiry

date), as they may have been oxidised or peroxidised, which can make them allergenic, or even carcinogenic in certain cases.

- Cat owners should be particularly careful, as cats are very sensitive to essential oils. This is not just because of their highly developed sense of smell (meaning that essential oils can overload their vomeronasal organ, making them apathetic or aggressive), but also because cats do not secrete the enzymes which are used to break down and eliminate the phenolic substances contained in essential oils, which they could ingest by licking surfaces which have been cleaned using products containing essential oils, for example. This could cause toxic hepatitis.

These precautions should be observed when using both household cleaning products and cosmetic products which contain essential oils. Similarly, essential oils should never be used by the following people:

- individuals who have a known allergy to an essential oil or one of its components;
- pregnant (risk of miscarriage) or breastfeeding individuals;

- children under 30 months, as a build-up of essential oils in the central nervous system can cause poisoning;
- children who have suffered any epileptic seizures or febrile convulsions in the past;
- individuals who suffer from asthma, as essential oils can irritate the respiratory system and trigger an asthma attack;
- individuals who suffer from epilepsy;
- individuals who have a G6PD deficiency (favism) should avoid methyl salicylate-based (gaultheria or wintergreen) and menthol-based (peppermint) essential oils, because they could cause anaemia (red blood cell deficiency) or jaundice if absorbed.

<u>Good habits</u>

When purchasing essential oils, get into the habit of checking the label.

Choose essential oils which are 100% pure, natural, organic and complete, meaning that they contain all of the oil's aromatic properties and have been extracted without the use of synthetic solvents.

Check that they are EOBBD (Essential Oils

Botanically and Biochemically Defined, meaning that the plant's Latin name, the part of the plant that has been used, the chemotype and the country of origin are all indicated on the label) approved, as this seal guarantees the essential oil's quality and combats fraud.

WHAT ARE ESSENTIAL OILS?

Essential oils are not oily bodies of fat as their name suggests, but rather the totality of active organic compounds found in aromatic plants. They are made up of a mixture of concentrated chemical components which have a variety of different active functions, including antiseptic, antibacterial, anti-inflammatory, deworming, antispasmodic and revitalising properties, depending on the essential oil in question.

The chemical composition of essential oils varies depending on the method used to extract them, as well as the plant's harvesting season and the ecosystem it grows in (altitude, exposure to sunlight, humidity, etc.). These are known as chemotypes, and refer to the dominant, biochemically active molecules contained in essential oils. It is important to be familiar with these chemotypes, as two different chemotypes from the same plant will have different therapeutic effects (and toxicity levels). For example, green myrtle (Myrtis communis CT 1.8 cineol) is a stimulant, whereas red myrtle (Myrtis communis CT myrtenyl acetate) has powerful antispasmodic properties.

THE HISTORY OF ESSENTIAL OILS

Humankind has been aware of the therapeutic properties of aromatic plants for millennia. The Aboriginal people of Australia used certain plants for healing purposes as early as 40 000 years ago.

The Egyptians mastered the art of distillation during antiquity (4500 BCE) and used it to isolate perfumes. These perfumes were used during courtship, but also held a great deal of religious significance (for example, they were used as part of the process for embalming corpses). The Egyptian distillation process involved soaking the plants in boiling water and then drying them by hand, and the perfumes were usually applied to the skin in the form of ointments and salves.

In Mesopotamia, the Persians (4000 BCE) also mastered the art of distillation and fumigation. Burning plants produced water vapour which contained the plant's active components, purifying the air and allowing the essential oils to be inhaled. For example, a room could be disinfected by boiling eucalyptus leaves.

Although the use of essential oils was initially limited to perfumes, it later became common in the medical sphere, where its use carried significant religious connotations. Essential oils were considered a way of prioritising the treatment of the patient's spirit rather than their body, and a way of preparing the dead to meet their maker.

Essential oils have also played an important role in traditional Chinese medicine (since 2800 BCE), and the earliest known written work describing recipes based on essential oils was allegedly written by the mythical emperor Shennong. This work is actually believed to be a compilation of ancient wisdom which had initially been passed down orally before being written down, but the original text has been lost and reconstructing it would be impossible.

The Inca, Maya and Aztec civilisations also used medicinal plants for healing, religious rituals and domestic purposes.

The Greeks (circa 300 BCE) used oils as perfume,

and Alexander the Great (king of Macedonia, 356 BCE-323 BCE) discovered their medicinal properties after his conquest of Egypt. The Greeks also strongly associated essential oils with religion, because according to Greek mythology, the oils were discovered by the gods. Hippocrates (Greek physician, 460 BCE-370 BCE), Aristotle (Greek philosopher, 384 BCE-322 BCE) and Theophrastus (Greek philosopher, 371 BCE-288 BCE) all wrote texts on the use of medicinal plants.

The Romans (150 BCE) also used essential oils, notably as perfumes and for religious purposes.

AHEAD OF HIS TIME

The physician Dioscorides, who was born in the 1st century in a Roman province in modern-day Turkey, wrote a text in Greek (though it is better known by its Latin name, *De Materia Medica*), which was considered a point of reference in European and Muslim pharmacology right up until the Renaissance.

Throughout the Middle Ages, monks and the nobility were generally the only people who were able to acquire essential oils. They were a crucial element in the search for the panacea, a mythical universal remedy which could grant immortality, and because it was believed that doctors had to treat their patients' souls in order to be able to heal their bodies, monasteries became centres of medical knowledge. In fact, religious authorities banned the use of perfumes for secular purposes. As a result, women who used herbs and who were knowledgeable about medicinal plants were believed to be witches, because according to the beliefs of the time, anyone who knew the secrets of healing must also have destructive powers.

Avicenna (980-1037) was a Persian physician and philosopher who discovered a method of distilling aromatic plants in order to extract the essential oils they contain in their purest form, and also invented the alembic (a distillation vessel). Later, in the 12th century, European forces discovered this invention during the Crusades and introduced the use of the alembic to their homelands.

During the 16th century, coils were used to cool steam, replacing the wet cloths and sponges which had previously been placed on top of alembics. From then on, the use and prescription of pure essential oils became common.

It was not until 1928 that René-Maurice Gattefossé (French chemist, 1881-1950) coined the term "aromatherapy". Although his research into essential oils proved that they can be used effectively for medical purposes, they never received the recognition they deserved. Bear in mind that synthetic molecules also began appearing at this time, and that the effectiveness of essential oils was falsely played down by pharmaceutical corporations.

In 1964, Jean Valnet (French doctor, 1920-1995) repopularised phytotherapy (medical treatments based on plant extracts) and aromatherapy among doctors and the public. He was the first to suggest dosages for essential oils.

PRODUCTION METHODS

Essential oils are extracted from aromatic plants. These plants account for approximately 10% of plant species, and synthesise active aromatic substances using secreting cells which can be found in different parts of the plant (flowers, leaves, roots, fruit, etc.).

There are many different methods of extracting essential oils, including steam distillation, dry distillation, cold pressing, enfleurage and solvent extraction. Essential oils which are suitable for use in aromatherapy can only be extracted via steam distillation and cold pressing, because these are the only methods which produce pure essential oils without altering their chemical composition. Essential oils which are produced using enfleurage and solvent extraction are used for perfumes.

Generally speaking, yields are tremendously low: several kilogrammes of plants are needed in order to produce a tiny bottle of essential oil, so essential oils can be very expensive.

<u>**P**OLLUTED **ESSENTIAL OILS**</u>

Always seek out organic essential oils, because any pesticides or other chemical fertilisers which were applied during the cultivation process will be absorbed by the water vapour during the distillation process, and will be concentrated in the essential oils. However, organic essential oils will not be contaminated with these chemicals.

STEAM DISTILLATION

Variations of this process have been used since antiquity, but the method we use nowadays was refined by Arab cultures.

The necessary parts of the plant are placed on a dish inside the alembic. Steam passes over this dish, causing the plant cells which contain essential oils to burst. The oils evaporate in the heat and, along with the water vapour, they pass through a cooling coil and condense into liquid. A distillate composed of essential oil and water can then be collected in an essencier. The water and the essential oil can then be decanted to separate them. The distillation water which is obtained through this process, which is known as the "hydrolat", can also be used in perfumes or in food.

Steam distillation at low pressure (1000-5000 Pa) and at a maximum temperature of 100°C is the extraction method which best conserves the properties of essential oils.

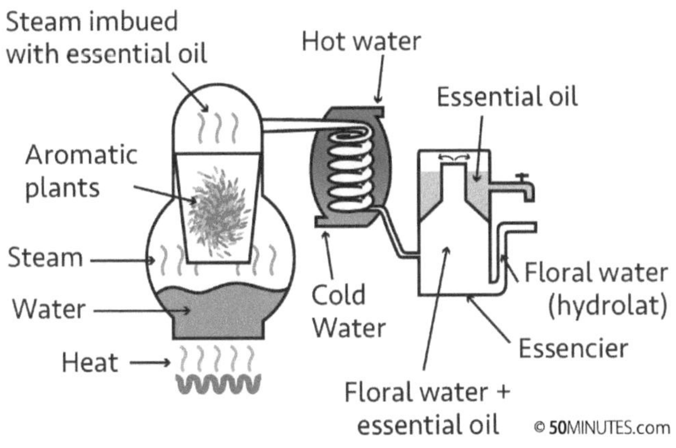

| Steam distillation

COLD PRESSING

This technique is used to extract the essential oils contained in citrus peel, and was first used in Sicily and Calabria in Italy in the 19th century.

The "pockets" of essence contained in fresh peel are burst using compression or abrasion techniques, which allows the essential oils to be collected. These oils are not pure, and contain wax and other non-volatile active substances, as well as other plant matter. This means that in order to extract the pure essential oils, you will have to centrifuge, filter and decant the solution.

DID YOU KNOW?

Although we now use the term "essential oils" for the product of distillation or cold pressing, it used to be known as "essence". Today, the term "aromatic essence" only refers to the active liquid secreted by aromatic plants. These terms were changed because the aromatic molecules contained in plant essences undergo certain changes during the production of essential oils through processes like oxidation and hydrolysis.

AROMATHERAPY

The term "aromatherapy" literally means "treatment through smell" and refers to healing techniques which incorporate the use of essential oils.

Aromatherapy is a holistic technique, which is based on the idea that any treatment should treat the entire human body. This means that they address our physical, psychological and emotional needs equally (which for some people also encompasses their mental and spiritual needs in the broader sense).

There are several different types of aromatherapy:

- symptomatic aromatherapy, in which essential oils are used to treat a symptom or illness;
- general aromatherapy, which considers the person as a whole and in which the essential oil is chosen with the aim of bringing the local or global imbalance which is causing the illness back into harmony with the rest of the body;
- aromatology, in which essential oils are used

to improve wellbeing outside of a medical context (massages, baths, skin treatments, etc.).

Generally speaking, it is important to pay attention to the way that the essential oils are applied, as the different methods of application correspond to different needs, and different safety measures are required for each one.

- **Dermal absorption.** This is the preferred method, because your skin and tissues can absorb the essential oils due to their lipophilic nature. In order to prevent dermal burns, they should be diluted using a vegetable oil base (sweet almond, argan or olive oil, etc.), especially phenolic essential oils. Never use more than the recommended doses:
  - dermal application: 4 to 5 drops of essential oils for children, or 6 to 10 drops for adults, which should always be mixed with 2 tablespoons of vegetable oil;
  - massages: mix 100 ml of vegetable oil with every 50 to 100 drops of essential oils;
  - in a bath: dilute approximately 20 drops of essential oils in a tablespoon of a neutral base for the bath; the bath should be no hot-

ter than 38°C in order to prevent scalding, and should last between 10 and 20 minutes;
   ◦ in cosmetics: mix 1 to 2 drops of essential oils into a dollop of your cream, shampoo or body lotion.
- **Respiratory absorption.** This method involves breathing in essential oils using an adapted diffuser, sprays released into the air, tissues infused with a few drops of oils, or by inhaling the vapour from a bowl of hot water.
   ◦ wet inhalation: place 2 to 3 drops of essential oils into a bowl of hot water, 3 times a day;
   ◦ dry inhalation: place 2 to 3 drops of essential oils on a tissue or on your handkerchief;
   ◦ diffuser: use 5 to 10 drops of essential oils, and use it for a maximum of 10 to 15 minutes so as not to oversaturate the atmosphere.
- **Oral ingestion.** This method is only suitable for certain essential oils (such as rosemary, lavender, peppermint, bergamot, lemon, basil, and so on), but it allows a very accurate dosage to be prescribed. It is therefore imperative to adhere to the recommended dosage. The drops of essential oil can be added to foodstuffs such as sugar, honey, yoghurt, vegetable oil or a neutral pill in order to avoid damaging the

lining of your throat and stomach. However, the best approach is to add the essential oils to gels prepared by a chemist. Many chemists also stock various items which contain essential oils and are specially designed to be orally ingested with no caustic side effects. The recommended dosage varies according to age:
  ◦ for adults: 2 drops of essential oils per dose, 3 to 4 times per day;
  ◦ for children under 7 years old: 1 drop of essential oils per dose, 3 times per day.
- **Other internal methods** (under medical supervision):
  ◦ mouthwash and gargles: the solution should be well diluted (1 to 5%) in 80% ethanol;
  ◦ suppositories and ovules: the final concentration of the essential oils should be between 3 to 5%, and they should be prepared by a chemist.

USING ESSENTIAL OILS IN AROMATHERAPY

Essential oils can be used in aromatherapy for a variety of purposes:

- to purify the atmosphere through their anti-septic, antibacterial, antiviral, acaricide and fungicide properties;
- to alleviate a variety of symptoms, such as ENT infections (rhinitis, colds, flu, seasonal allergies, etc.), digestive problems, etc;
- to improve sleep quality and to help you fall asleep more easily;
- to combat stress and its symptoms (fatigue, insomnia, anxiety, back pain, etc.);
- to alleviate muscle and joint pains;
- to alleviate headaches and migraines;
- to treat skin damage through their anti-scarring, anti-inflammatory and antiseptic properties;
- to combat lice;
- to repel mosquitoes;
- to improve wellbeing through massages and skin treatments, etc.

BOOST THE EFFECTIVENESS OF ESSENTIAL OILS

It is possible to create so-called "essential oil synergies" using aromatherapy. The term "synergy" can be used to refer to either a mixture of essential oils with complementary therapeutic properties which have more powerful effects when used in combination, or a mixture of essential oils with similar properties which are more effective when used together.

ESSENTIAL OILS USED IN AROMATHERAPY

Bergamot (*citrus bergamia*)

- **Properties:** antiseptic, antispasmodic, digestive, sedative.
- **Uses:**
  - lack of appetite and digestive problems;
  - gut infections, colitis, flatulence, constipation;
  - sleeping problems, restlessness;
  - acne, eczema, itching;

- ◦ greasy hair.
- **Methods of application:**
  - ◦ oral;
  - ◦ dermal;
  - ◦ atmospheric diffusion.

Bitter orange (*citrus aurantium*)

- **Properties:** antibacterial, antifungal, antispasmodic, painkiller, anxiolytic, immunostimulant, anti-scarring.
- **Uses:**
  - ◦ improving sleep;
  - ◦ stress, anxiety;
  - ◦ skin infections;
  - ◦ cramps and muscle contractions;
  - ◦ coughs;
  - ◦ digestive problems;
  - ◦ greasy hair.
- **Methods of application:**
  - ◦ oral (under medical supervision);
  - ◦ dermal;
  - ◦ inhalation;
  - ◦ atmospheric diffusion.

Camphorwood (*cinnamomum camphora*)

- **Properties:** antiviral, antibacterial, antifungal, anti-inflammatory, expectorant, immunostimulant, tonic, spasmolytic.
- **Uses:**
  - respiratory infections;
  - gastroenteritis;
  - herpes, shingles;
  - muscle contractures;
  - arthrosis, rheumatism;
  - fatigue, recuperation.
- **Methods of application:**
  - oral (under medical supervision);
  - dermal;
  - inhalation;
  - atmospheric diffusion.

Chamomile (*chamaemelum nobile*)

- **Properties:** antispasmodic, digestive, tonic, painkiller, anti-anaemic, febrifuge, deworming, emmenagogue, relaxant, anti-scarring, anti-inflammatory.
- **Uses:**
  - easing digestion;

- ◦ regulating periods;
  - ◦ combatting stress, improving sleep and making it easier to fall asleep;
  - ◦ irritated skin, especially dry or aged skin;
  - ◦ dermal inflammations, pain, headaches;
  - ◦ lightening blond hair.
- **Methods of application:**
  - ◦ oral (under medical supervision);
  - ◦ dermal;
  - ◦ inhalation;
  - ◦ atmospheric diffusion.

Cinnamon (*cinnamomum verum*)

- **Properties:** antiseptic, antibacterial, anti-parasite, antifungal, antispasmodic, tonic, cardiac and respiratory stimulant, immunostimulant.
- **Uses:**
  - ◦ bacterial or viral infections;
  - ◦ general fatigue;
  - ◦ muscle aches, cramps;
  - ◦ infected wounds, insect bites;
  - ◦ stimulating the cardiovascular system.
- **Methods of application:**
  - ◦ oral (under medical supervision);
  - ◦ dermal;
  - ◦ atmospheric diffusion.

Clary sage (*salvia sclarea*)

- **Properties:** antiviral, antibacterial, anti-inflammatory, antispasmodic, antiperspirant, calming, phlebotonic, euphoria-inducing, stimulant, cellular regeneration.
- **Uses:**
    - problems related to the menopause, painful periods, irregular menstrual cycles;
    - sleeping problems;
    - cramps and muscle contractions;
    - bowel spasms;
    - skin problems;
    - gingivitis;
    - regulation of perspiration.
- **Methods of application:**
    - oral;
    - dermal;
    - atmospheric diffusion.

Clove (*eugenia caryophyllus*)

- **Properties:** antiviral, antifungal, antibacterial, painkiller, numbing, anti-scarring, calming, sedative.
- **Uses:**
    - gut, urinary and lung infections;

- ◦ toothache, minor oral sores;
  - ◦ easing digestion;
  - ◦ constipation;
  - ◦ physical and intellectual stimulant.
- **Methods of application:**
  - ◦ oral (under medical supervision);
  - ◦ dermal;
  - ◦ mouthwash;
  - ◦ inhalation;
  - ◦ atmospheric diffusion.

Eucalyptus globulus

- **Properties:** antiseptic, antibacterial, antiviral, antifungal, decongestant, cooling, insect repellent.
- **Uses:**
  - ◦ clearing breathing passageways;
  - ◦ bronchial and lung infections;
  - ◦ urinary infections;
  - ◦ thrush;
  - ◦ preventing and treating rhinitis, bronchitis, angina, laryngitis, and colds.
- **Methods of application:**
  - ◦ oral (under medical supervision);
  - ◦ dermal;

- inhalation;
- atmospheric diffusion.

Eucalyptus radiata

- **Properties:** antiviral, antibacterial, antifungal, anti-parasite, anti-inflammatory, cough suppressant, expectorant, immunostimulant, energising.
- **Uses:**
  - treating infections in the upper respiratory system;
  - flu;
  - coughs;
  - treatment for herpes, urinary infections and thrush;
  - for a general boost after winter.
- **Methods of application:**
  - oral (under medical supervision);
  - dermal;
  - gargling;
  - atmospheric diffusion.

Gaultheria (*gaultheria procumbens*)

- **Properties:** anti-inflammatory, painkiller, analgesic, spasmolytic, rubefacient.
- **Uses:**
  - cramps, contractures, muscle pains;
  - lumbar pains, sciatica;
  - joint pains, rheumatism, polyarthritis;
  - tendonitis.
- **Methods of application:** dermal.

Grapefruit (*citrus paradisi*)

- **Properties:** antiseptic, antiviral, antibacterial, antifungal, antidepressant, liver detoxification, diuretic, cardiotonic, immunostimulant, antioxidant.
- **Uses:**
  - digestive problems;
  - depression;
  - elimination of toxins;
  - water retention;
  - cellulite;
  - cooling;
  - combatting bad smells and air purification.
- **Methods of application:**
  - oral (under medical supervision);

- dermal;
- atmospheric diffusion.

Helichrysum (*helichrysum italicum*)

- **Properties:** antiviral, antibacterial, anticoagulant, anti-bruising, anti-inflammatory, antispasmodic, anti-scarring, dermocosmetic properties.
- **Uses:**
  - bruising;
  - venous insufficiency, capillary fragility, varicose veins;
  - cold sores, acne, dermatitis, stretch marks;
  - wrinkles.
- **Methods of application:**
  - oral (under medical supervision);
  - dermal.

Lavandin (*lavandula hybrida abrialis*)

- **Properties:** calming, relaxant, sedative, anti-stress, spasmolytic, painkiller, anti-inflammatory, anti-bacterial.
- **Uses:**
  - mild depression;
  - migraines;

  - insomnia and sleeping problems;
  - skin infections, wounds, burns, sores;
  - cramps and muscle contractions.
- **Methods of application:**
  - oral (under medical supervision);
  - dermal;
  - atmospheric diffusion.

Lavender (*lavandula angustifolia*)

- **Properties:** sedative, anxiolytic, painkiller, local anaesthetic, anti-inflammatory, anti-infection, antifungal, anti-parasite, anti-scarring, hypotensive, spasmolytic.
- **Uses:**
  - insomnia and sleeping problems;
  - stress, irritability;
  - migraines;
  - difficulty concentrating;
  - problems related to the menopause;
  - head lice;
  - cramps and muscle contractions;
  - preventing infection of burns, wounds and stings.
- **Methods of application:**
  - oral (under medical supervision);

- ◦ dermal;
- ◦ inhalation;
- ◦ atmospheric diffusion.

Lemon (*citrus limon*)

- **Properties:** antiseptic, antiviral, antibacterial, antifungal, invigorating, cleansing, anxiolytic, anti-anaemic, slimming.
- **Uses:**
  - ◦ anaemia;
  - ◦ fatigue, memory problems;
  - ◦ ENT or lung infections;
  - ◦ digestive or liver problems;
  - ◦ travel sickness;
  - ◦ circulation problems;
  - ◦ air purification;
  - ◦ mosquito repellent.
- **Methods of application:**
  - ◦ oral;
  - ◦ dermal;
  - ◦ atmospheric diffusion.

Lemongrass (*cymbopogon winterianus*)

- **Properties:** antiseptic, anti-infection, anti-fungal, anti-inflammatory, anti-rheumatic,

anti-parasite, antispasmodic, mosquito repellent.
- **Uses:**
  - skin infections (acne, fungal infections);
  - insect bites;
  - bowel spasms;
  - easing rheumatism, joint pains, arthritis, tendonitis;
  - mosquito repellent.
- **Methods of application:**
  - oral (under medical supervision);
  - dermal;
  - atmospheric diffusion.

Niaouli (*melaleuca quinquenervia*)

- **Properties:** antiviral, antibacterial, antifungal, anti-parasite, anti-inflammatory, expectorant, decongestant, mucolytic, anti-scarring, insect repellent.
- **Uses:**
  - respiratory infections;
  - viral infections;
  - urological infections;
  - gynaecological infections;
  - skin problems;

- insect bites;
- sunburn;
- prevention of radiotherapy burns.
- **Methods of application:**
  - oral (under medical supervision);
  - dermal;
  - inhalation;
  - atmospheric diffusion.

Peppermint (*menthe piperita*)

- **Properties:** painkiller, antiviral, antifungal, anti-inflammatory, antispasmodic, vasoconstrictive, tonic, antioxidant.
- **Uses:**
  - respiratory infections;
  - gastro-intestinal problems;
  - nausea;
  - travel sickness;
  - difficulty concentrating;
  - skin irritation and itching;
  - herpes, shingles;
  - sunburn;
  - muscle aches;
  - headaches.

- **Methods of application:**
  - oral (under medical supervision);
  - dermal;
  - inhalation;
  - atmospheric diffusion.

Rose geranium (*pelargonium graveolens*)

- **Properties:** antiviral, antifungal, anti-inflammatory, anti-scarring, firming, draining, insect repellent.
- **Uses:**
  - gut, urinary and lung infections;
  - fungal infections;
  - water retention, cellulite, excess weight;
  - preventing stretch marks;
  - excessive perspiration;
  - burns, eczema;
  - insect bites.
- **Methods of application:**
  - oral (under medical supervision);
  - dermal;
  - inhalation;
  - atmospheric diffusion.

Rosemary (*rosmarinum officinalis*)

- **Properties:** antiviral, antibacterial, anti-inflammatory, cardiotonic, decongestant, expectorant, diuretic, stimulant, digestive.
- **Uses:**
  - joint pains, rheumatism;
  - muscle cramps;
  - easing digestion;
  - diarrhoea;
  - respiratory infections, flu;
  - headaches;
  - fatigue;
  - stimulate memory and concentration;
  - hair loss.
- **Methods of application:**
  - oral (under medical supervision);
  - dermal;
  - inhalation;
  - atmospheric diffusion.

Scots pine (*pinus sylvestris*)

- **Properties:** anti-inflammatory, antibacterial, antiviral, anti-neuralgic, respiratory antiseptic, expectorant, decongestant, diuretic, toning, painkiller, percutaneous, insecticide.

- **Uses:**
  - respiratory infections;
  - flu;
  - rheumatism and muscle pains;
  - urinary infections;
  - painful periods;
  - circulatory problems;
  - fatigue, asthenia, overwork, recuperation.
- **Methods of application:**
  - oral (under medical supervision);
  - dermal;
  - inhalation;
  - atmospheric diffusion.

Sweet orange (*citrus sinensis*)

- **Properties:** antibacterial, antiviral, antifungal, calming, sedative, anti-stress, choleretic, cholagogue, anti-nausea, regulation of digestive problems, purifying, deodorant.
- **Uses:**
  - anxiety, stress, insomnia;
  - heart palpitations;
  - easing digestion and the expulsion of bile;
  - improving appetite;
  - insect bites;

◦ purifying and scenting the air.
- **Methods of application:**
  ◦ oral (under medical supervision);
  ◦ dermal;
  ◦ atmospheric diffusion.

Tea tree (*melaleuca alternifolia*)

- **Properties:** antiseptic, antibacterial, antiviral, antifungal, anti-parasite, anti-inflammatory, antioxidant, anti-scarring, immunostimulant.
- **Uses:**
  ◦ bacterial or viral ENT and respiratory infections (sinusitis, angina, bronchitis, flu, ear infections), urinary infections (cystitis), vaginal infections and mouth infections (gum disease, canker sores);
  ◦ acne, abscesses, cold sores, fungal infections, psoriasis, insect bites;
  ◦ greasy hair, head lice.
- **Methods of application:**
  ◦ oral (under medical supervision);
  ◦ dermal;
  ◦ inhalation.

Ylang-ylang (*cananga odorata*)

- **Properties:** antibacterial, antifungal, anti-inflammatory, antioxidant, anti-stress, cardiovascular regulation, anti-scarring, painkiller.
- **Uses:**
  - palpitations, irregular heartbeat, hypertension;
  - stress, anxiety, depression;
  - sleeping problems;
  - infected wounds;
  - acne;
  - insect bites;
  - patients in intensive care on morphine.
- **Methods of application:**
  - oral (under medical supervision);
  - dermal;
  - atmospheric diffusion.

TREATING MINOR AILMENTS

Common cold

Pour six drops of one of the following essential oils (or two drops each of three of the following essential oils) into a bowl of boiling water: *eucalyptus globulus*, *eucalyptus radiata*, lavandin, lavender, niaouli, peppermint, rosemary, scots pine, tea tree. Breathe in the steam for about five minutes.

Occasional headaches

Use your index fingers to massage one drop of peppermint essential oil into your temples and the nape of your neck, taking care to avoid your eyes.

Fatigue

Add one drop of lemon essential oil to a teaspoon of honey and take this mixture three times a day, between meals, for two to three weeks.

Rheumatism

Pour some vegetable oil (arnica, hazelnut, grape, olive oil, etc.) into the palm of your hand. Add one drop each of lavender, ginger and (if the pain is very severe) gaultheria essential oils, then massage the affected joints.

Burns

Apply one or two drops of lavandin essential oil

to the burn two or three times a day.

Cold sores

Apply one or two drops of tea tree essential oil several times a day as soon as the first symptoms appear.

Bruises

Apply two drops of helichrysum essential oil as soon as possible after receiving the blow, and reapply every ten minutes without exceeding six drops. Alternatively, massage well with a mixture of 10% helichrysum oil and 90% arnica oil and reapply several times a day as needed. Caution: never apply to an open wound.

Pimples

Apply one drop of tea tree essential oil to each pimple three times a day.

HOUSEHOLD REMEDIES FOR IMPROVED WELLBEING

For a deep-cleansing facial

Pour three cups of boiling water and four drops of essential oil into a large bowl:

- ylang-ylang essential oil for dry skin;
- calendula essential oil for normal skin;
- peppermint essential oil for oily skin.

Lean over the bowl, keeping at least 25 cm away from it at all times. Cover your head with a towel and breathe in the steam for five minutes. Rinse with fresh water.

Relaxing facial lotion

Pour five drops of lavender essential oil and 5 cl of sweet almond oil into an opaque glass bottle (so that the essential oil does not lose any of its potency through exposure to sunlight). Shake the bottle before use.

To tame thick or unruly hair

Pour one or two drops of rosemary essential oil

into the palms of your hands and apply to your hair.

To lighten blond hair

Add 30 drops of chamomile essential oil to a bottle of neutral shampoo (or two drops to a dollop of shampoo). Apply the shampoo and leave for 5 to 15 minutes, depending on how much lighter the desired shade is. Rinse thoroughly.

Deodorant spray

Mix 100 ml of floral water (witch hazel or orange blossom) and 40 drops of the essential oils of your choice in a spray bottle.

For example:

- 100 ml witch hazel, 20 drops lavender essential oil, 10 drops tea tree essential oil, 10 drops lemon essential oil;
- 100 ml orange blossom, 20 drops rose geranium essential oil, 15 drops clary sage essential oil, 5 drops lemongrass essential oil.

Most importantly, the resulting fragrance should be pleasant. Shake well before each use.

Homemade Eau de Cologne

Add the following to an opaque glass bottle:

- 150 ml alcohol at 70° proof (or vodka);
- 100 drops bergamot essential oil;
- 50 drops lemon essential oil;
- 50 drops lavender essential oil;
- 30 drops neroli essential oil;
- 10 drops rosemary essential oil.

Leave for six months before using, keeping it out of direct sunlight.

A NATURAL HOME

Living in a healthy, clean environment is something we all aspire to. You can make your own cleaning products at home using natural, biodegradable substances, which allows you to stop using the toxic products that are responsible for domestic pollution, which causes allergies, headaches and respiratory problems such as asthma.

Essential oils are a key ingredient in these products, as they fragrance them and help to purify our homes. Here are some simple products you can create, as well as a list of essential oils which you can use around your home on a daily basis.

MULTI-PURPOSE CLEANING AGENT

Mix 300 ml alcohol vinegar, 150 ml water and 1 tsp *eucalyptus radiata* essential oil in a spray bottle. This can be used to clean stainless steel sinks, kitchen countertops, modern surfaces, etc. Spray and rub with a soft cloth; there is no need to rinse.

FLOOR CLEANER

Mix the following in a 2 l container:

- 0.75 l black soap (cleans and disinfects);
- 0.5 l linseed oil (adds shine, nourishes wood and saturates tiles);
- 0.5 l water;
- 30 drops tea tree essential oil.

Shake before use. Use one or two dashes of the mixture per bucket of hot water.

LIQUID DETERGENT

- For whites, mix the following in a 3 l container:
    - 35-40 g Marseille soap shavings (depending on the desired consistency of the detergent);
    - 3 tbsp sodium bicarbonate;
    - 1 l very hot water.

Mix and leave to stand for one hour, then add 1 l lukewarm water and 10 drops lemon essential oil to fragrance. The next day, add 1 l cold water then shake. Use 100 to 200 ml of the mixture per laundry load.

- For colours, replace the sodium bicarbonate

with 3 tbsp washing soda, as this will brighten the colours in the clothes.

FABRIC SOFTENER

Pour a cup of white vinegar or a quarter of a cup of sodium bicarbonate and a few drops of lavender, lemon, eucalyptus or rose essential oil as fragrance into the washing machine tray.

Mix the following in an empty bottle of fabric softener with a measuring cap lid:

- 1 l alcohol vinegar;
- 0.5 l distilled water;
- 10 to 20 drops tea tree essential oil.

Shake before use. Pour one or two capfuls into the fabric softener compartment depending on your water hardness.

AIR FRESHENER

Pour a few drops of essential oils into a cup of water and set it on top of a radiator, or add five to ten drops of essential oils to a diffuser, depending on the model.

To create your own homemade blend of fragrances, mix the following in an opaque glass bottle:

- 60 ml alcohol at 70° proof (or vodka);
- 20 ml distilled water;
- 10 drops lemon essential oil;
- 10 drops sweet orange essential oil;
- 10 drops grapefruit essential oil;
- 10 drops lavender essential oil.

Leave to soak for at least two weeks, keeping it out of direct sunlight. Shake occasionally before spraying.

MOSQUITO REPELLENT

- Mix 10 drops of lemongrass essential oil and 10 drops of rose geranium essential oil in a diffuser.
- Mix equal amounts of lemongrass and rose geranium essential oils in an opaque spray bottle and spray on clothes, blankets, curtains, etc.

WOOD MAINTENANCE

Mix the following in a small spray bottle:

- 5 tbsp lemon juice or vinegar;
- 5 tbsp olive oil;
- 15 drops lemon essential oil.

Spray on the surface which needs maintenance then rub with a soft cloth.

Essential oil	Properties
Cinnamon (*cinnamomum verum*)	• antiseptic, antibacterial, antiviral, antifungal, anti-parasite
Clove (*eugenia caryophyllus*)	• antibacterial, antifungal, anti-parasite, antiviral
Eucalyptus (*eucalyptus globulus; eucalyptus radiata*)	• antiseptic, antibacterial, antiviral • clean fragrance
Fir (*abies balsamea*)	• antiseptic • clean fragrance
Grapefruit (*citrus paradisi*)	• airborne antiseptic

Essential oil	Properties
Lavender (*lavandula spica*)	• antiseptic, antibacterial, antiviral, antifungal, mothproofing • clean fragrance
Lemon (*citrus limon*)	• antiseptic, antibacterial, antiviral • clean fragrance
Lemongrass (*cymbopogon winterianus*)	• antiseptic, antibacterial, insect repellent
Peppermint (*menthe piperita*)	• antiseptic, antibacterial, antiviral, antifungal, deworming • clean fragrance
Pine (*pinus sylvestris*)	• antiseptic • clean fragrance
Tea tree (*melaleuca alternifolia*)	• antibacterial, antifungal, anti-parasite, antiviral
Thyme (*thymus vulgaris*)	• antibacterial, antiviral, anti-parasite

| Summary of household uses

Humans have always sought to discover the many benefits of aromatic plants. Over time, we have learned how to extract, distil and use essential oils for healing, as perfumes, to improve our wellbeing and to clean our homes. Nowadays, essential oils play a crucial role in natural medicine, wellbeing and daily household cleaning.

However, they can be somewhat dangerous. This means that it is important to apply them using the appropriate methods, doses and precautions in order to prevent accidents and to get the most out of them. To do so, you will need to familiarise yourself with them, by speaking to chemists and herbalists who have training in this area and can give you informed advice, by reading books on aromatherapy, or even by attending one of the increasingly common workshops for beginners, which give participants the chance to learn about a few essential oils and how they can be used to improve you and your family's health and wellbeing.

Essential oils can also be extremely useful for household cleaning, eliminating the need for complicated, expensive products. All you need are a few simple, environmentally-friendly products which you can use to make your home a healthier environment.

FAQS

HOW SHOULD ESSENTIAL OILS BE STORED?

Essential oils should be stored in a dark place, between 5 and 30°C, in a bottle which should be kept upright (because the oils can damage the lid if the bottle is left in a horizontal position). Once the bottle has been opened, make sure that you close the lid again properly, because essential oils are volatile and oxidisable. You should also check the expiry date. Any mixtures of essential oils and vegetable oils that you have prepared yourself should only be kept for a maximum of six months, because vegetable oils turn rancid very quickly. Most importantly, make sure to keep them out of the reach of children.

WHAT IS THE DIFFERENCE BETWEEN ESSENTIAL OILS AND VEGETABLE OILS?

Essential oils are obtained from aromatic plants and have concentrated active properties, whereas vegetable oils are extracted from oleaginous plants (almond, hazelnut, sunflower seeds, wheat germ, argan, calendula, etc.) using cold pressing.

CAN ESSENTIAL OILS CAUSE ALLERGIC REACTIONS?

Yes, even though they are natural products. This sensitivity to essential oils affects 1-2% of the population, and generally involves dermal reactions. These allergies do not always manifest the first time someone comes in contact with an essential oil; the incubation period can be very long and it can take years for an individual to develop an allergy. As a precaution, it is recommended to test a small amount on the crook of your elbow and wait 48 hours to see if you have an allergic reaction before using a full dose.

Also bear in mind that certain essential oils (citruses) are photosensitising and can cause skin reactions when your skin is exposed to UV light. As such, you should use these oils in the evening and never while you are exposed to sunlight.

WHICH ESSENTIAL OIL SHOULD I BUY FIRST?

If you only buy one essential oil, make sure that it is lavender. It is an extremely versatile essential oil, which has antiseptic and anti-inflammatory properties and can also treat many minor daily ailments. It has relaxing effects and can be applied to any skin or hair type. It can also be used to fragrance your home and linen.

HOW SHOULD I REACT TO AN ACCIDENT?

- If any essential oil accidentally comes into contact with someone's eyes or mucous membranes, use a vegetable oil (olive, peanut, wheat germ, etc.) to rinse the irritated area and solubilise the essential oil.
- In cases of inhalation, take the victim out of the room so that they can breathe in some

fresh air.

- If an essential oil is ingested accidentally, do not induce vomiting; contact your doctor or a poison control centre.

When speaking to your doctor or the poison control centre, make sure to mention:

- the type of essential oil used and the amount that was consumed;
- the type of exposure (ingestion, skin contact, eye contact, inhalation, etc.);
- whether or not the essential oil was diluted with a vegetable oil, for example;
- the time that has elapsed between the accident and the call being made;
- the symptoms;
- the victim's age.

It may be necessary to have your stomach pumped or to undergo treatment in a hospital. There is no specific antidote for essential oils, and treatment is based on the symptoms.

WHERE CAN I BUY ESSENTIAL OILS?

Nowadays, essential oils can be found in many places, not just chemists and drugstores; you can also buy them in specialised organic or nature and wellbeing shops, and also by ordering them online (though you should always pay careful attention to the terms of delivery). Finding a sales point which employs someone who specialises in aromatherapy is always the best approach, because you can ask them for advice if necessary and they will be able to ensure that the products sold in the shop are stored appropriately. Good aromatherapy requires good raw materials, meaning high-quality essential oils.

We want to hear from you!
Leave a comment on your online library
and share your favourite books on social media!

FURTHER READING

BIBLIOGRAPHY

- Angenot, L. (2012) *Les effets toxiques en aromathérapie*. Brussels: Société Scientifique des Pharmaciens Francophones.

- (2015) Aromathérapie. La Revue du Praticien – médecine générale. 946.

- Boisseau, N. (2009) *Le ménage au naturel*. Paris: Éditions Alternatives.

- Brossollet, J. (No date) Dioscoride Pedanius. Universalis.fr. [Online]. [Accessed 15 November 2017]. Available from: <http://www.universalis.fr/encyclopedie/dioscoride-pedanius>

- Charier, S. (2013) *Le guide pratique des huiles essentielles. 600 recettes pour soigner au naturel les maux du quotidien*. Issy-les-Moulineaux: Éditions Marie-Claire.

- Charrie, J. and Clermont-Tonnerre, M. (2013) *Ma santé au naturel toute l'année. Conseils d'un médecin pour toute la famille*. Paris: Éditions France Loisirs.

- Corbel, S. (2012) Aromathérapie et problems digestifs. Guide pratique à utiliser à l'officine. *Hippocratus.com*. [Online]. [Accessed 15 November

2017]. Available from: <https://www.hippocratus.
com/modules/mdc_Conseils/conseils_fiche.
php?CodeRubrique=&CodeService=&ModeCons-
eil=6&Rub_Page=1&id=851&id=851>

- Foit, M. (2014) *Aromathérapie de A à Z avec des plantes qui poussent en France*. Kindle.

- (No date) *Guide d'utilisation des Huiles Essentielles Bio et Chémotypées Green For Health*. Aix-en-Provence: Éditions Green For Health.

- (No date) Historique des huiles essentielles. *Néroliane.com*. [Online]. [Accessed 15 November 2017]. Available from: <http://www.neroliane.
com/neroliane-guide-historique>

- (2007) Huiles essentielles. Tableau par plantes. *Herbessence.ch*. [Online]. [Accessed 15 November 2017]. Available from: <http://www.herbessence.
ch/pdf/Tableau%20des%20huiles%20essentielles.
pdf>

- (2009) *Le guide de la maison au naturel*. New York: Sélection du Reader's Digest.

- (No date) L'histoire des huiles essentielles. *CompagniedesSens.fr*. [Online]. [Accessed 15 November 2017]. Available from: <https://www.compagnie-des-sens.fr/
histoire-des-huiles-essentielles>

- (No date) Raffa, le grand ménage. Raffa.grandme-nage.info. [Online]. [Accessed 15 November 2017]. Available from: <http://raffa.grandmenage.info>

ADDITIONAL SOURCES

- Lawless, J. (2014) *The Encyclopaedia of Essential Oils: The Complete Guide to the Use of Aromatic Oils in Aromatherapy, Herbalism, Health & Well-being*. London: Harper Thorsons.

- Worwood, V. A. (1997) *The Fragrant Mind: Aromatherapy for Personality, Mind, Mood and Emotion*. London: Bantam.

50MINUTES.com

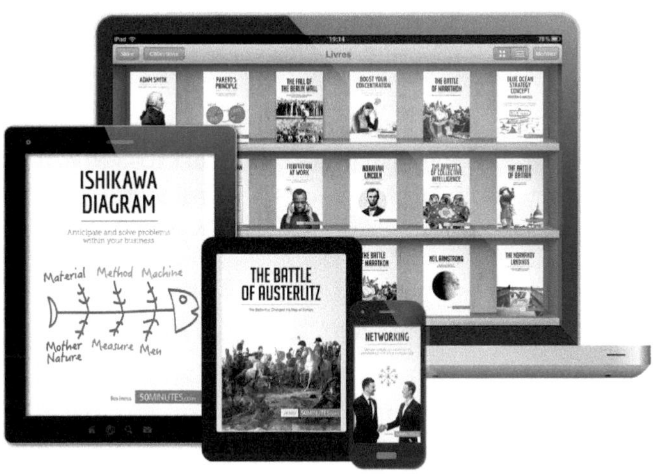

IMPROVE YOUR GENERAL KNOWLEDGE

IN A BLINK OF AN EYE !

www.50minutes.com